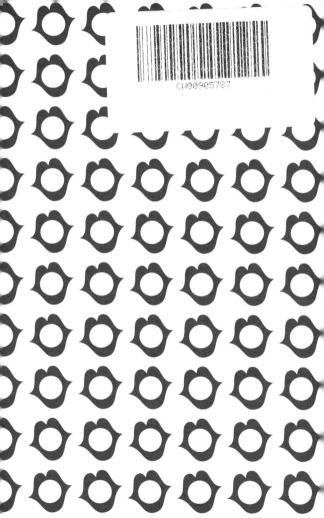

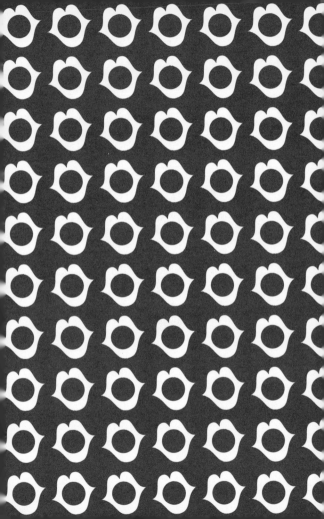

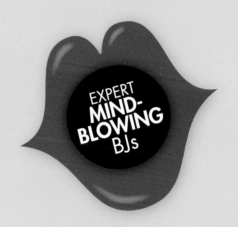

EXPERT
**MIND-
BLOWING**
BJs

THIS IS A CARLTON BOOK

This edition published
by Carlton Books Limited
20 Mortimer Street
London W1T 3JW

10 9 8 7 6 5 4 3 2 1

ISBN 978 1 84732 808 3

Printed and bound in Italy

Senior Executive Editor: Lisa Dyer
Managing Art Director: Lucy Coley
Designer: Gülen Shevki-Taylor
Production: Kate Pimm

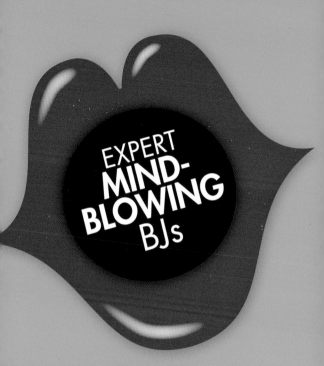

EXPERT MIND-BLOWING BJs

LISA SWEET

CARLTON
BOOKS

CONTENTS

Introduction

There are all kinds of ways to go down on a guy. You might use a slow, sweet and sensual style; others times your mood may be passionate, profound and powerful. All are good. You will never hear a guy say he has had a bad blowjob. But what really makes him rise to attention is when the giver doesn't just bob her head up and down his penis as though her head is on a spring. Sure, that will produce the goods, but there's a difference between adequate and amazing.

This book is all about how to lick your man into a frenzy. Even if you feel you give really fine fellatio already, it's guaranteed you will find something in these pages that will further blow your man's mind.

Section One

REFRESH IT

Fact: Every man loves blowjobs. Even
if you're not the world's greatest, if he's getting
a blowjob, he's pretty much already on Cloud
Nine. That's not to say there's no wrong way
to give head, because there is. But if his dick
is in your mouth, for him things are already off
to a great start.

There are many technical aspects that come into play, but even the most experienced, tongue-twisting mouth magic begins with mastering a few basic steps.

A few essentials you might want to have on hand before you begin: a drink of some kind to wet your whistle, lip balm to keep things slick, lube to keep things even slicker, and a hair band to hold your tresses away from your face so he can have a clear view of the action.

Head Start

Read on for a quick 1-2-3, blow-by-blow
refresher course on how to give a great lip.
Use separately, or put them all together to
make him want to twist and shout.

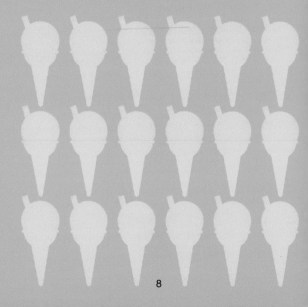

Get into it

Enthusiasm cannot be overemphasized. Giving good head means you give good face. The thing is, only half of what makes a blowie perfect is technique. So no matter how raunchy your routine is, it's going to seem ho-hum if you don't put some joy into your moves. If you treat oral sex like a chore, well, then it's definitely going to suck – in a bad way. If you want to give a guy an excellent blowjob, show some zeal. Don't just dive into the job headfirst. Look at his goods with the same desire you would a chocolate chip cookie dough ice-cream cone. He wants you to relish it, crave it, savour it.

REFRESH IT: Let him know you like it by softly moaning as you take him into your mouth. Remember there is a person attached to that penis – look up and make eye contact occasionally. And don't work in silence. A good blowjob makes loud, gross suction-y noises. So don't be afraid to slobber all over his love muscle. It should be as wet and sloppy as possible, especially during your power move. If the slurping noises make you self-conscious, crank some tunes to mask the mouth ruckus. Just make sure you can keep the beat!

Get into position

You'd be surprised what difference a slight change of angle can make when it comes to sensation – for you as well as him.

There is no way you are going to be able to show him your love if you aren't physically comfortable. Fellatio can put a lot of pressure on your neck and jaw. Lying down, facing each other is probably the most comfortable position for both of you.

REFRESH IT: You can curl your body so that you can determine the depth and angle of his thrusting. Also, let him slide one of his legs between yours so you can rub up against him.

Channel your inner porn star and sink to your knees in front of him while he remains standing. This will give you the wide range of motion needed and plenty of access to his package without the strain.

REFRESH IT: Switch it around so you are working him from behind – this way you can trail your tongue around his entire package.

If you want to control his action, have him on his back and crouch between his legs.

REFRESH IT: Straddle him and bring your boobs into play. With gravity on your side, it'll be easy to envelop him in your cleavage by simply leaning forward and undulating a little.

Get going

Be a little unpredictable. Alternate between sucking, stroking, squeezing, slurping and swirling.

Try using just your mouth: This is the best start if he isn't completely flexing his muscle. Put his entire penis in your mouth while you suck and lick. Hold off on moving your mouth up and down until he's at least partially erect. Another mouth-only move for a not-yet-but-soon-to-be erect penis is to repeatedly suck and swallow, allowing for his entire penis to be in your mouth.

REFRESH IT: Don't just open your mouth and close it around his cock. Slide it in. Once your lips have a firm hold, suck in small pulses, using ever increasing pressure (and if you are worried it's too hard, have him suck your finger to show you how strong he likes his suction). It will feel like he has landed in a warm, wet, snug vagina.

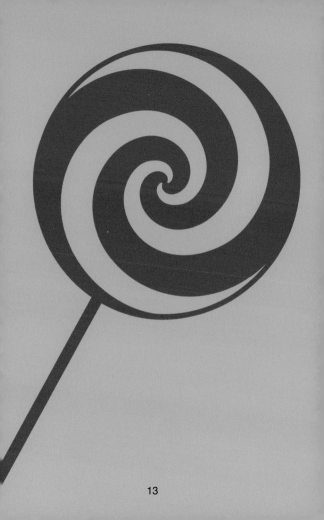

13

Give him some tongue: There's a reason it's called "giving head". Pay particular attention to his ultrasensitive tip. Lick it like a lollipop. Swirl your tongue around the sensitive spot underneath the ridge of the head.

REFRESH IT: You can simulate deep-throating by switching between flicking his tip with your tongue and gliding your mouth up and down the shaft. A firm hold is good, but don't suck it too tight. Also, be sure you've got him wet like a slip and slide, with water-based lube or spit, so that friction doesn't get in the way of fun.

Give him a hand: Your hands can be remarkably useful – they add variety, they can play with other parts and they can make up for whatever you can't take into your mouth. Placing one hand at the base of the penis with the thumb and forefinger circling the shaft, will help to keep him erect and in position. Now make the same ring with the thumb and forefinger of your other hand, but use this one against your lips to follow the movement of your mouth up and down. Hands can be particularly useful if you find yourself about to gag – let your hand do the work and give yourself time to recover before going back down. This is also "handy" if he is on the XL side. But make sure you add lots of juice so your hand will slide easily up and down instead of just catching on his dry skin.

REFRESH IT: Do the twister. When you slide your hand up his shaft, twist your wrist. A twisting motion gets you into a smoother rhythm than the straight up and down. Synchronize your mouth and hands so you are sliding your hand up and down on the base of his cock in beat with your mouth moving up and down on the rest of it.

- Another good trick is to wrap your hand around the top of his cock and put your mouth over your hand. Then, slide your hand down the shaft and your mouth down on top of it in a fluid motion until your hand meets the base of his cock. It will feel like you're sliding your mouth all the way down him even if you can't.

BALL PLAY

Don't forget to have some fun and games with his balls. Just use a lighter touch than you would with his main equipment.

Fondle them while you suck his cock.

Lightly pull them away from his body and lick the soft sensitive skin underneath.

Lick one while cupping the other in your hand. Gradually take the entire ball into your mouth, then alternate between licking it directly with your tongue and juggling it in your mouth.

Put both in your mouth by using one hand to circle the top of the sac and gently pull it down to bring the balls together into a neat swallowable package.

The Complete Instructions to His Privates

They don't come with an owner's manual, so here is the ultimate instruction manual for turning on and using his favourite power tool. Caution: best operate when fully wet.

Meatus: This opening in the tip of the penis (where his lava flow starts) quivers when poked with a stiff tongue.

Corona: This is the slightly raised ridge that separates the head from the shaft (not always visible until he's erect if he's not circumcised), and is a seam of sizzle when treated to long, languorous licks.

Frenulum: Although just a tiny bud of skin on the underside of the penis where the folds and head come together, it is easily the most sensitive spot on his penis and many men may come too quickly when it receives too much attention. To make him whimper, place the tip of your finger on it, then take his shaft and your finger into your mouth. As you move your mouth up and down, rub your finger over the F-spot.

Shaft: Since the actual shaft doesn't have many nerve endings, sucking up and down on it is going to do little more than keep him in a holding pattern. The trick is to concentrate on a hot spot at the base, near where it meets the balls. To hit a home run, suck hard while his bat is in your hands.

Testicles: Extremely sensitive to any stimulation. All it takes to make him melt is to very gently suck them into your mouth.

Perineum: It's not strictly on his tool, but think of it as a must-have accessory. Pressing this ultra-sensitive area between his testicles and bottom hole with your tongue or fingers can actually help keep him hard longer.

The Big Gulp

Giving him a suck down and then skipping the swallowing part once he ejaculates is like cheering on your favourite athlete in a race and then leaving before they cross the finish line. You have put a lot of effort into giving him pleasure. Now see it through to the end. Luckily, swallowing can be as easy as 1-2-3. Here's a refresher on how to drink him down to his last drop. Cheers!

Know when he is about to blow

Recognizing when he is getting close keeps you in control of his flow. The signs are the same every time – the head of his penis will swell slightly, his hips will probably start thrusting forwards and then a few tiny drops of clear liquid will drip from the penis tip.

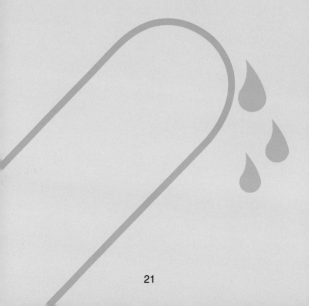

Stop the flow

Lots of guys don't always want the BJ to be their big finish. Instead, they would rather you treat it like foreplay.

If he does want to go all the way, you need to decide: swallow, sip or spit? Whatever your choice, start to suck harder and pump your head faster. Don't even think about slowing down.

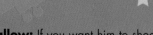

Swallow: If you want him to shoot, open your mouth wide and let him hold his torpedo and squeeze it. He'll be more accurate than you, lowering the chance of a miss and splatter.

REFRESH IT:
Once he's finished,
look him in the eye as
you envelope him with
your mouth and suck to
wring him dry. Open
wide to show him
you're done.

Sip: If you can't swallow the whole shot at one time, just press the penis a little bit to control the speed. This way, you can aim it towards your inner cheek and hold it there to swallow in small amounts. If it's the taste that turns you off, pool the semen in the front of your mouth, far from the parts of your tongue that register bitter salty flavours, and then swallowing quickly in one gulp.

REFRESH IT: To kick things up a notch, press your thumb against the base of his penis so the tube the semen flows through is blocked. At the same time, suck vigorously on the head. This will delay the flow for a few deliciously long moments, giving you time to prepare where you want it to shoot and him time to whimper with delight.

Spit: Since running to the bathroom is not an option (unless you are doing it next to toilet), try cutting down on "the load" so there's less to deal with, by placing a fist between his balls and his bottom and pressing hard just as he is about to come. You can also make not swallowing so sexy that he will want you to do it all of the time. You can let him spill over your breasts and then rub it into your skin, licking your fingers. Or let him come in your mouth and instead of swallowing, let it trickle out of your mouth and all over him.

REFRESH IT: Do it in the shower – he'll love the sensation of the warm water cascading over him and never notice that you just let his essence dribble down the drain.

The Director's Cut: An uncircumcised man still has his foreskin (the soft flap of skin covering the head of the penis when it is not erect). Once he's locked and loaded, the foreskin rolls back on its own and works just like its circumcised bro. But until then, that hoodie on his penis head is a pleasure centre chockablock with tingly nerves. This is where you can really work your magic, because the foreskin is ultrareceptive to every touch, movement, temperature change, massage and grip that comes its way. Of course, that extreme sensitivity also means you have to be more careful about teeth and hand pressure. As a rule of thumb (or penis), it is always better to start too soft and gradually build up. If he screeches like a girl, you probably went too far. Read on for three ways to have fun with his foreskin.

Hold the skin in place over the head with your lips and oh-so-lightly nibble. Then push your tongue up under the head, swirling it around the underside of the foreskin and over the head. You can always place your hand on the shaft if you need help keeping the skin covering the head.

Push the skin off the glans with your lips, licking at the frenulum as you go.

Insert your tongue into the foreskin and circle around the head with it. You can also use your fingers to gently massage the head through the foreskin, alternating with deep tongue licks.

Caution: Check under his hood! Uncircumcised penises need that extra scrub, so lift up the foreskin and get some scent-free soap under there! Otherwise it gets Smegma bacillus build-up (dick cheese, the waxy white substance secreted by the penis glands, aka gross).

Section Two

EXPERT BLOW-JOB TRICKS

The average penis does not seem like such a complicated thing to please: simply suck it here, lick it there and don't forget to show a little gung-hoism and chances are, he will explode. But what lifts a common-or-garden variety blowjob into the realm of extraordinary are a few smooth moves. Well, take a deep breath, oral-sex-goddess-in-training. What follows is the start-to-finish on eight penis pleasing BJ scenarios – all guaranteed to make you go down in his memory as the best he ever had (to the point that he'll get a rise in his pants when he hears a name sounding even remotely like yours). Follow each one point-by-point or pick and choose for your (and his) pleasure. Drum roll please…

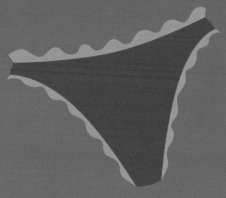

Top Twenty Tips

1

To get him excited, take charge and grab the initiative. Undress him and run your fingers gently over the underside of his penis.

2

Look into his eyes – it brings the experience to a whole new level, plus he loves to watch!

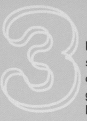

3 If he's not fully at attention, start with simple licking and then take his penis gently into your mouth. Don't suck or blow at first.

4 Deeply kiss the V-shaped lines of muscle that run down a man's pelvic area, from his hips to his groin, before moving on to the main course.

Make sure he's well-lubed. If you're worried about taste, use an edible, flavoured lube; otherwise saliva will keep him wet and slippery.

6 Heat up edible lube in your mouth and then slowly dribble the hot fluid over his penis.

7 Cover your teeth with your lips and keep your lips firm.

8 Gently massage his balls. Don't squeeze, as the testicles are highly sensitive.

To intensify his orgasm, press
against his perineum with your
thumb, moving it in tiny circles
– or try two fingers for two
seconds and then release.

9

10 Wrap your hands around
whatever part of the penis you can't
take into your mouth and move up
and down simultaneously with your
mouth – this will feel as though
you're taking in the whole penis.

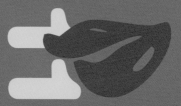

Switch between mouthing and licking. Alternate between deep sucks and light, teasing ones.

12

Use your hand and fingers at the same time as your mouth, lips and tongue.

13

Using a flicking action with your tongue, back and forth over the head of the penis, will really get him going.

14 Run the flat of your tongue from underneath his balls to the tip of his penis several times in quick succession.

15 Rub the head of his penis over your face and lips.

16 Get good vibrations. Humming while he's inside your mouth will send vibrations down his shaft, or alternatively hold a vibrator to your cheek.

17 Once he's close to climaxing, stop varying your moves and keep a steady rhythm.

18 Breathe on his cock, then blow gently with your hot breath.

19

Listen to your man and gauge his reactions – what works for one man may not work for another.

20

Remember the five key elements to a good blowjob: warmth, wetness, eagerness, repetition and at least one surprise manoeuvre.

The Perfect BJ

Blow his mind with a long, hard suck.

Best Position: Him lying flat on his back with his legs spread and you kneeling down in front of him. You will need to fully support yourself with your legs, because you will be using both of your hands throughout.

Mouthwatering Tip: Leave the lights on. He wants to see and appreciate your handy (and mouth) work.

The key is to start
from the top and take
it slow. Think of it as blowjob
foreplay. Suck his fingers to give
him a taste of what's on the menu.
Slowly kiss your way down his chest,
stopping at the nipples (about 50 per cent
of guys love having their nubs played with,
and the other half didn't know they did
because no one ever gave their nipples
that much TLC before). Trail your
tongue down his belly
to between his legs.

At the same time, use
your hands to rub, squeeze
and caress him from his neck all the
way down to his thighs and bottom and
back up again. With each pass, increase the
pressure and begin lingering in his sensitive
places, like the inside of his thigh, his waist,
his upper shoulders and the back of his neck.
Eventually, leave your hands below his belt. Take
his penis in your hands and test its heft. Really
feel it. Run your fingers, palms and then your
whole hand up and down his shaft. Do this
a few times, increasing the pressure
with each rubdown. Make it
obvious you just want to eat
him up.

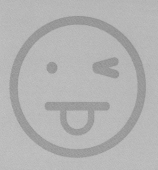

Sure, this builds the pressure but it also gives you a sense of what makes his toes curl. Read his body – does he prefer it when you give some love to the top or bottom of his shaft? (Rarely does a man like both equally well.) Is the head of his penis more sensitive than the corona or frenulum? If you're not sure, check his face – is he in a happy shiver-me-timbers place or does he look like he is about to yawn?

Start
your
mouth
moves by
holding his penis
in your hand and slow
kissing and licking just the
head. Catch him off balance by
slipping the entire thing (if you can) in
your mouth. This has the double purpose of
sending a jolt of pleasure right to his groin
while making him slick and easy to work with.
Slip him out and lick his now slippery pole,
but this time going all the way up and
down the shaft. The wetter it is, the
better, so don't be afraid
to slobber.

Now you're ready to move on and suck him up. This will feel more intense than just moving your mouth up and down his shaft. As you pull him back out of your mouth, leave the head of his penis in and continue stroking and sucking until you go back down. If he pops out, just start at the base again.

Don't worry if you can't fit all of him in your mouth. Actually, the less you stuff in, the more you can do. Use your hands to make up the difference – just grasp him around the base and stroke.

There is no law that says: A blowjob means that the mouth must remain in contact with his penis at all times. So keep things interesting with the following moves. There is no particular order, and the more you mix it up, the more interesting it will be for him:

- Flick your tongue across the head of his penis as you suck it.

- Swirl your tongue around his shaft as you suck up and down.

- Switch between mouthing it and licking it.

- Make eye contact.

- Give him a deep, loving kiss.

- Alternate between deep sucks and quick little teasing ones.

- Rub or lick the patch just behind his balls.

- Blow warm air against his shaft.

- Don't forget his balls – check out Ball Play on page 17.

- When he's ready to blow, pull your head back so that just the head is between your lips while pressing your tongue against the underside. This way, he gets maximum pressure and you don't get drowned in jism.

- Or you can skip all of the above and buy him one of the "Mouth" series for his birthday. This ultimate in boy sex toys has a vibrating orifice that mimics the warm pressure of a perfect blowjob.

The Quickie BJ

This one is perfect for advert breaks during Match of the Day. Master this and you will make him come in under two minutes. Quickie BJ's are also a good way to restart his engine once he's already blown a gasket.

Best Position: You want him to have a lot of control with this move to keep the action speeding along at a high pace, so sit with your legs straight out in front of you while he kneels and straddles your hips. This way he will be able to cup your head. If you need a bit more breathing space, try leaning back a bit.

Mouthwatering Tip: Keeping your tongue in the action at all times during this BJ is key.

To get a guy off as quickly as possible, lock your lips at the base of his cock and, sucking hard, move your mouth up and down the bottom three-quarters of his shaft (just estimate – men don't like rulers near their tools) at a quick, steady pace while pressing your flattened tongue against the underside of his penis. Be sure to jack up the pressure with both your lips and tongue. That's it. If you can keep this up with a steady pace for 120 seconds, you can both go back to watching the match without missing a thing.

However... there are a few flourishes you can throw in to keep him revved. Because the coronal ridge is the most responsive part of his engine, any tooling around there will keep him over the speed limit:

Place your lips around the head and twirl your lips wetly and gently around the ridge.

Suck hard on the tiny profusion of flesh (think goldfish mouth moves).

Tap your tongue gently against the coronal ridge while using your hand to crank his shaft.

SPEED HIM UP

Blowjobs can occasionally be a lot of work (hence the "job" part!). If you want to speed things up, try these tricks.

- Zone in on his frenulum. Packed with nerve endings, it's a big, no-fail Big-O trigger. With every lick, add a little extra tongue pressure in that one spot until he climaxes.

- Wrap your thumb and index finger around the shaft, about 2.5 cm (1 inch) above the base, and pull down while sucking down on the head.

- Launch sequence still not happening? Give up and make him come another way – try switching to hand action or via intercourse. Save face by sighing, "You made me so hot I can't wait to feel you inside me."

- Getting Lift Off? If his penis swells, his body tenses and his balls draw close to his body, he's gonna blow. Instantly recall what he does with his body during his intercourse orgasms – does he start jackhammering or stay slow and steady? Mimic that action with your mouth.

The Miss
Destiny Desire BJ

Give head like a pro – a pro-stitute, that is.

Best Position: Lie on the bed, with your head just over the edge, so that your head is somewhat tilted downward. This will open up your throat to allow for deep penetration (read on for why that's important with this BJ). Control his movements by placing your hands on his pelvis.

Mouthwatering Tip: Do this later in the day when it's easier to control your gag reflex.

Why is a man willing to pay for a BJ? Two words: Deep throating.

Unfortunately, the average length of your oral cavity is about three and a half inches while the average penis measures in at around five and a half inches. You do the math.

This is why it rarely works when he grabs your head at the crucial moment and shoves. You need to prepare to swallow his sword or your gag reflex will kick in. First, slather him with lube – either your own saliva (use your imagination) or a flavoured lube, chocolate syrup, ice cream or anything that you have a craving for. Once he's nice and wet, hold him in your hands and take him s-l-o-w-l-y into your mouth.

Smother the impulse to take a deep breath before you go deep. Instead, exhale and switch to breathing through your nose. This way, you will make room for as much as three more of his inches (which is probably all you'll need).

Direct the tip so that
it is resting against
the roof of your mouth.
Pause to open your throat
by using the same movement
that you would if you were chugging down a drink.
At the same time, use the base of your tongue to
gently push him down your throat. Start humming
– it will feel amazing to him and help keep your
gag reflex at bay. Remember to keep breathing
through your nose.

It will take a few times before you can do this in
one smooth motion, so practise (he won't object!).

Once he's in, there are a few things you can
do to make him hotter than a forest fire:

• Contract your throat muscles to make him feel
like he's being milked

• Swallow a few times – the sensation will make
him reel.

Backup plan: If this is
too much for you to swallow
at once, you can perform a "fake"
deep throat. While you're taking him
in deeper, flatten your tongue vertically
until his penis hits it. This will appear to
alter the depth of your mouth and he'll
think you've got him further back than
he's used to. You can keep him further
distracted by layering your lips in
ultrabright red gloss and keeping
on a pair of stilettos.

Deep Throating Tips

Blame the movie, but no man feels his life is complete unless he has been deep-throated. The problem is that the average throat is not made for swallowing a 6–8 inch (yes guys – that really is the standard measurement) sausage whole.

- Lie back on the bed and hang your head off the edge. He can then stand by the side (on pillows if necessary) so that his penis is lined up with your mouth.

- Pay attention to the angle of the dangle – work from above with an up-curving penis and below with a down-pointing one.

- If you gag easily, point him slightly towards the side of your throat instead of straight down. He won't go in as deep, but he'll never notice the difference.

- Stop and relax your throat muscles every 1.5 cm (½ inch) or so before letting him go deeper.

- Swallow – when he tickles the back of your throat, that is. It will help gag your gag reflex and widen things.

The Make It Up BJ

Giving great head means you never have to say you're sorry.

Best Position: He's lying down and you are on top, totally in control.

Mouthwatering Tip: Mount your defense from a position of power by cuffing and blindfolding him before having your wicked way.

Twelve things you can do to him that will have him begging you for mercy:

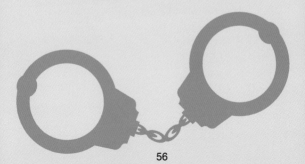

1
Tease him until he's ready to combust. Head south with your mouth but pass on by with just a hot breath. Repeat a few times before taking him in your mouth in one smooth gulp.

2 Let him in only halfway, alternating shallow and deep sucks in a way he can't predict.

3 While nibbling on his shish kebab, slip a well-lubed finger inside his bottom hole and wiggle it around. You're stimulating his prostate, a hot spot that, when pressed, makes him prostrate with pleasure.

4 Trace a figure eight with your tongue over his balls. Flick your tongue lightly and quickly, barely touching them, as you go round and round his sac.

5 Roll his glans (head) in your mouth while stroking his shaft up and down and massaging his testicles. You may need to prop him up afterwards.

6 Suck his glans as hard as possible, as if you're drinking from a straw and you've hit the bottom of the glass. To add some extra oomph, flick your tongue quickly over the tip of his shaft with each inward suck.

7 With his penis loosely in your mouth, slowly shake your head as if you were saying "no". Make sure his shaft hits all the corners of your mouth.

8 A variation on no. 7: keeping his penis in your mouth, move your head in a circular clockwise, then counterclockwise motion.

9 Add your tongue to the mix and flick it across the head of his penis while you're circling or shaking your head.

10 Hold his penis in your hand. With your mouth wide open, stick out your tongue and gently slap the bottom of his shaft against it, aiming so you hit the frenulum. The vibrations will send shivers up his spine.

11 Slipping on a pair of finger vibrators will turn your blowjob into a whoa! job.

12 Swallow, sucking him dry.

The Break-Up BJ

If you can't make it up, at least give him something to remember you by – swallow him deep. Sucking hard, squeeze his balls with one hand and grab his shaft with the other, and jerk him off while deep throating him. Hold his juice in your mouth and slide up to give him a last, lingering kiss – letting his semen drain back into his mouth as you do.

The Tasty BJ

These simple, scrumptious steps will have you feasting on his pickle.

Best Position: When bringing food to your BJ blowout, it's best if he lies flat to keep his utensil from making a mess.

Mouthwatering Tip: Keep a towel nearby to clean up afterwards.

One of the biggest concerns about heading south of the border on a guy is that his downtown won't smell or taste good. While you want to watch out for DDD's (Dangerous Dirty Dicks), some guys are an acquired taste. There are studies that show what he chows down on during the day shows up in his sweat scent. What goes in, comes out, literally. Unfortunately, the surest way to a nicer tasting carrot, is clean living. But if your guy is addicted to his vices, here are some samplers to sweeten the pot:

Suck on a strong mint or mentholated cough drop immediately before giving head. You'll add zing to your mouth work and kill any sour tastes. A dab of toothpaste on his balls will add a tingle, but steer clear of mouthwash or breath sprays, as they may contain alcohol, which can sting.

Drinking mint tea heats up your mouth, which can increase sensation and blood flow to his penis

Flavoured lubes and sprays will keep things sweet and juicy.

Pour on the Champagne. The bubbles will give him a heady tingle.

Just before going down on him, pop some crushed ice cubes in your mouth. The dual sensation of the ice and the heat of your mouth will be a huge turn on, and the sensation of the crushed ice can add depth to your mouthwork while giving his naughty bits a quick rinse (especially helpful if his member wears a turtleneck).

Turn him into a sweet treat by holding slightly warm hot fudge in your mouth before you eat him up. The thick texture will give him a sexy, smooth sensation.

Tossing some Pop Rocks candy into your mouth works just like a DIY vibrator.

Slip your favourite fruit Lifesaver (Polo) into your mouth before heading for his buoy – it will create more saliva and you can use the shape to tease him, slipping it over the head of his penis and sucking hard.

Mix him a pineapple and cranberry juice – the citrus contains natural acids that may counteract against the alkalinity or bleachy taste of his splunk, making him taste sweeter. For best results, repeat daily for a month.

The Two-Timer BJ

To give is fine, but to receive (at the same time) is divine!

Best Position: Lying on your sides, head to toe.

Mouthwatering Tip: Suction isn't just for BJs. It's easy to get distracted when giving and receiving at the same time. Having him switch up his moves and sucking hard on your clitoris will give you the focus you need.

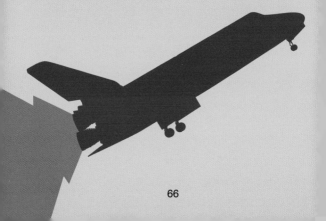

This move is harder
to do than deep-throating.
To master this ultimate pleasure, work
yourselves up with plenty of individual
foreplay first, so you are not depending on
in-sync slurping to send you into the stratosphere.
Then, as you both lick, let your hands massage
each other's booties – there are large muscles
there, so rubbing them will make for an
even greater release.

Just don't get so caught up in the Zen of
harmonized hoo-hah that you lose out on your
own bliss moment. If you gotta blow, let it go. He'll
catch up. And vice versa. If he's prone to post-
carnal coma, hand him a vibrator and tell him
to turn it on in case of emergency.

The On-Location Blowjob

Everything you need to know to give blow-to-go – anywhere but in the bedroom.

Best Position: Each location has its own specific pose, but the all-purpose on-the-go BJ stance is one where he is standing or sitting and you are kneeling or crouching in front of him.

Mouthwatering Tip: These BJs are not for long, lingering lovefests – you want to get in quick, do the job and be reapplying your lipstick within five minutes tops, so suck it to him with plenty of hard, pulsating pressure.

Under the table: Ensure there is a long tablecloth to hide your hijinks from view. Slide between his legs and nibble his corn on the cob. Use the table napkin to clean up any spills.

In the car: BJWD (Blowjobs While Driving) are not covered by insurance. Best to pull over to a shoulder or rest stop to lick his joystick. Because you are working from the side, it will be easier to weave with a lot of head bobs than maintain a steady speed.

In the bathroom at a party or on an airplane: Make use of the spigot. Wet your hands to juice things up quickly. Kneeling in a bathroom is not recommended, and you probably don't want to get your mouth anywhere near the bog, so try crouching in front of him and using your hands to squeeze things along.

At the office: Have him sit back with his butt on the edge of a chair or desk, legs apart, and then kneel between them. Take dictation by spelling letters with your tongue all over his keyboard.

Washing Machine: Add a buzz to your blow and have him hop on top of the washer during the spin cycle. Lean on his thighs as you bob over him so you don't end up with a sore back.

In a closet at his parents', the shower, a lift (elevator) or a changing room:

More blood rushes to the pelvic region while a man's on their feet, resulting in a firmer erection and ultimately a much more intense orgasm, so this should be fast, furious and fabulous. As you kneel in front of him, suck hard on the tip and circle the base of his stick with your finger and thumb, squeezing slightly to increase the pressure of his explosion.

The Birthday BJ

Surprise party not included.

Best Position: Polls reveal that his hands-down favourite BJ position is you kneeling in front of him and him standing, holding your head.

Mouthwatering Tip: A BJ in any shape or form is the perfect gift.

1

Wake him with a morning treat.

Take advantage of his morning salute. The key is not too much pressure or too fast to begin with or you may accidentally trigger his fight or flight reflex and end up with his foot in your face. If he is sleeping on his tummy, spoon against him and reach around to his goods and caress. He should roll over. If not, just give him a push to put him in position – he is not going to complain about you waking him before the alarm!

Even More Mouthwatering Tip: If you have a strong gag reflex it will be worse in the AM, so switch this to a sleepy-bye BJ instead.

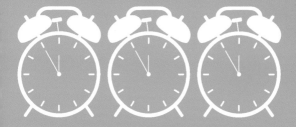

Stud him.

A tongue piercing is overrated unless you know how to use your tongue. The key is not too much, but not too little. Use your tongue on the back of his digit and around the head. Start slowly at the top like you're making out with it, then work your way down and increase the speed. Concentrate on rubbing against the sensitive underneath bits for a titillating touch.

Even More Mouthwatering Tip: If you use a light touch, you may be able to pull this off with a fake removable tongue ring.

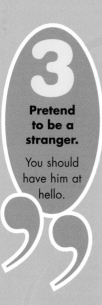

3

Pretend to be a stranger.

You should have him at hello.

4

Dom him.

You're usually both so focused on pleasing each other, that neither of you get to bask in being a sex object. So take the reins. Tell him you are going to tie him up and blindfold him to have your wicked way with him until he can't stand up for a half an hour. Or else skip the small talk – just grab him, roll him into position and give him the oral affection he deserves.

Even More Mouthwatering Tip: Let him play King O' The Mattress – and grab your head, push you down and tell you exactly what to do to him.

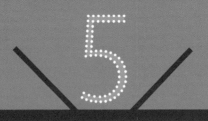

Give him a game-winning blow-by-blow.

Time your moves to the action on the telly.
Pick up the pace so he scores at the same
time as his team. Cover your ears as he
screams, GOOOOOOOOOOOAAAAAAAA
AAALLLLLLLL!

Even More Mouthwatering Tip:

Make sure he has a bowl of snacks and
a beer before you start.

6

Feast his eyes.

You probably already know that guys are extremely visual, but it can be hard for him to get a decent view while you're down there lavishing his penis with love. Place a standing mirror next to you so he can check you out. The combo of feeling and seeing you will blow (pun intended) his mind.

7

Give him a pearl necklace.

He won't mind that you aren't swallowing if you let him make like a porn star and come all over your face.

Even More Mouthwatering Tip: Slip in some slapping. Pop him out and slap his big boy against your tongue or face a few times.

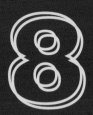

Give him an all-day sucker.
When you're planning a long trip downtown, you need to know how to cool his tool so he can last and last.

Chill his dill: Holding your lips tightly around him, go as far down on the shaft as you comfortably can. Now open wide and suck in a lungful of air while moving your mouth back up to his tip. With your mouth still open, exhale slowly through your mouth as you move down his pole again. Basically, you're cooling him on the upward stroke and heating him on the downward.

Slow him down: If his hips start bucking and you're not ready for his big finish, you can slow him down without pulling his emergency break by switching the sensation – use your hands to gently squeeze him or slide him between your breasts until he is back to cruising.

Even More
Mouthwatering Tip:

Sliding his big boy into a cock ring will keep him going strong. If you choose one that vibrates, he will become your boy toy for ever. Place the vibrating part so that it touches the balls to create a whole avalanche of sensation while you work magic with your mouth. Place it just over the shaft to focus the vibration on the scrotum, or just behind his balls to hit his hot spots.

Section Three

THE BIG FINISH

No argument: He loves when you go down on him and he loves it even more when you show that you love it too. But sometimes you might try something that he doesn't love. It doesn't matter if you are so orally skilled that you can tie his stem into a knot with your tongue. There are some things that you think are going to make him groan with gratitude and pleasure but actually makes him want to roll over and zip up his pants.

Or maybe the hitch is with his penis. Perhaps his favourite player isn't up for a command performance or, frankly, it is so badly behaved it shouldn't even be let out in public.

Luckily, you don't have to suck at going down on him – unless you want to! Many of these problems can be made better with a few small adjustments. Read on for quick fixes for your most common blowjob blunders.

Low Blows

You're doing your best, but things don't always go to plan. Here are the all-time classic blowjob blunders and how to make them right.

1 You're tooth torturing.

If he's moaning with pain, then you may be giving him too much dental friction.

👄 **SUCK IT UP:** Cover your teeth with your lips before biting down.

2 You're gagging.

Puking him up will put a damper in his rod.

🍃 **SUCK IT UP:** See The Miss Destiny Desire BJ on page 50–55 for how to deep-throat. Also, try holding him steady with your hand and breathing in instead of just holding your breath.

3
It's too soft.

He is not an ice-cream cone nor is he a clitoris. Guys' equipment tends to be tougher than womens', so feel free to manhandle.

🍃 **SUCK IT UP:** Make like a Hoover and suck – hard!

4
It's too dry.

Yes, he likes friction but at the same time, he also likes BJs that are sloppy wet – go figure.

SUCK IT UP: Keep a glass of H_2O nearby to wet your whistle and keep the juices flowing.

5
You think you have ESP skills (Extra Sensory Penis).

Not all BJs are created equal.

SUCK IT UP: Since he knows best what feels good to him, ask for feedback.

6
You're making him yawn.

Even a BJ can become same ol', same ol' if you never vary your style.

👅 SUCK IT UP:
Mix your moves up. If you usually suck, lick; if up and down's your standard range of motion, move side to side.

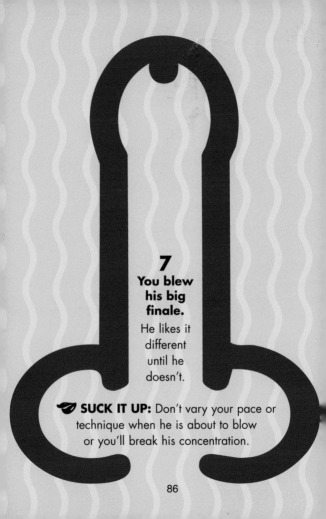

7
You blew his big finale.
He likes it different until he doesn't.

🌊 **SUCK IT UP:** Don't vary your pace or technique when he is about to blow or you'll break his concentration.

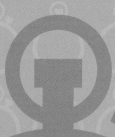

8
He blew his
big finale.

You know he likes it when he
comes early to the party.

SUCK IT UP: Give him 15 minutes
to rest and then start from the beginning.
He will be able to control himself this time
because he's already had his pleasure.
(Yes, he is having his cake and eating
it – but then, so are you!)

9 He's a keeper.
One of the worst things he can do while you're working his wood is take too long.

🦷 **SUCK IT UP:** Concentrate on his frenulum to bring forth a geyser.

10
He's Mr Softie.
Some men won't immediately stand to attention when you start.

🦷 **SUCK IT UP:** Lick the shaft and take it in your mouth and roll around it with your tongue. He'll start picking up his pace.

11
He spews over your hair or clothes.

Lightbulb! This is why you should keep a towel nearby. For now, clean up (think *Something About Mary* and pretend it's hair gel). Next time, try swallowing. Otherwise, pay attention when he is about to blow and aim it away from you.

12
You choke on his sausage.

Don't try to swallow more than you can chew. Instead, make him a manageable size. Use your hands to caress his base, or lay on your back with your head dangling to open your throat wide.

Poison Penises

What to do with a smelly, soiled or sick dick? Having unprotected oral sex is risky if your partner has herpes, genital warts, gonorrhea, chlamydia, syphilis or is HIV positive, whether you swallow or not. If you aren't sure about his best boy's bill of health, it makes sense to wrap it up before you give it an oral wash. Here's how to give him a Safe Sex BJ.

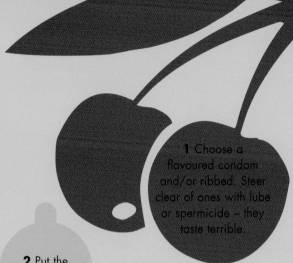

1 Choose a flavoured condom and/or ribbed. Steer clear of ones with lube or spermicide – they taste terrible.

2 Put the condom in your mouth with the reservoir tip pointing towards your throat, and the ring of the condom in front of your teeth (careful you don't snag it).

3 Press the reservoir tip against the roof of your mouth with your tongue. You want to keep the air out of the tip as the condom is going on.

4 Dab his tip with a smidgeon of lube to make the roadway smooth.

6 Lower your head and put the condom on his tip, squeezing the reservoir tip with your tongue against the head.

5 Wrap your hand around his base to keep things straight.

7 Cover your teeth with your lips and use your mouth to carefully roll the condom down the shaft.

Even More Mouthwatering Tip:

If he's just dirty or stinky (a common problem if he's collared), then suggest moving the action to the shower. You can wash him down with soap and water before completing the job with your tongue.

Boys' Toys

Anal beads/balls
These are put slowly into the anus and then pulled out rapidly during an orgasm to accessorize pleasure.

Butt plug
Short and slim, the plug has a flared end. It can help intensify orgasm and can also be used to prepare for anal sex.

Cock ring
Usually made from rubber, leather or metal, the ring goes around the base of the penis (and sometimes the testicles) to pump up his erection for longer than usual. There are vibrating versions available.

Lubricants
Emollients such as oils, lotions and creams that, when applied to the penis, skin or a sex toy can increase its slipperiness, making sex a more juicy affair.

Masturbation Cup
A vacuum cup that delivers a sucking "deep throat" sensation. It has a round head that completely covers the head of the penis.

Monkey Spanker
With a powerful vibrator in the handle, this is a disc of premium silicone. You insert the penis through the hole in the centre of the disc (after applying a liberal amount of lube).

Prostate Massager
Shaped and angled to provide pressure and stimulation on the prostate and surrounding area, this hands-free, vibrating massaging tool is a perfect introduction to "P-Spot" play.

Vibrator
Any toy that vibrates, usually with a choice of speeds. They come in every shape under the sun, from bullets to eggs. Slimline ones are good for holding against the perineum or testicles.

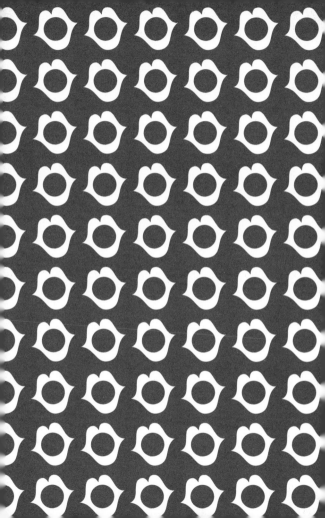

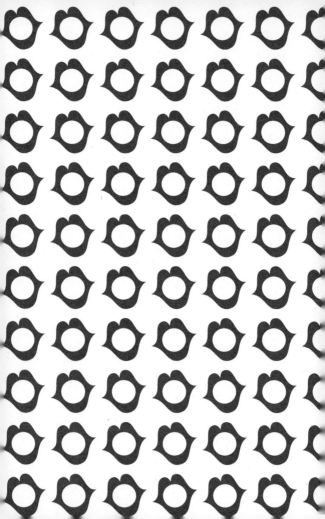